# YOU'RE NOT STUCK WITH HPV!

ROSA ROMERO

# YOU'RE NOT STUCK WITH HPV!

ROSA ROMERO

**DISCLAIMER**

This book has been written for informational purposes only, therefore it should be used only as a guide, but it does not replace in any way the medical or therapeutic treatment that you may need in difficult circumstances. In this regard, all readers are advised to follow the information mentioned herein at their own risk. The author and publisher shall have no liability to any person or entity with respect to any personal loss or damage caused or alleged to be produced directly or indirectly by the information contained in this book. All readers are advised to seek professional medical advice when they need it.

The purpose of this book is to convey the author's experience. The author and publisher do not warrant that the information contained in this book is completely complete and shall not be liable for any errors or omissions.

Copyright © **2021 Rosa Romero**

Title: YOU'RE NOT STUCK WITH HPV!

ISBN 978-1-365-67253-8

**All rights reserved**

No part of this book may be reproduced or stored in any system—electronic, mechanical, photocopying, memory storage, or otherwise—or transmitted in any form or by any means, without the express permission of the publisher.

# INDEX

INTRODUCTION ............................................................. 9
CONFUSION .................................................................. 11
WHAT YOU NEED TO KNOW ..................................... 17
WHAT YOU SHOULD DO ............................................. 23
FOODS THAT HEAL ...................................................... 29
GENITAL CARE FOR MEN AND WOMEN ............ 35
DON'T DESPAIR ............................................................. 43
THE FEARS ..................................................................... 47
DEFINITIONS .................................................................. 53

# Introduction

The human papillomavirus – hereinafter HPV – is a very common sexually transmitted infection, and 90% of people have it or will have it at some point in their lives.

Hello, my name is Rosa, I am not a health professional, I just wrote this book to share my experience with precancer HPV, stress, depression and everything that comes associated with the HPV virus. You got it? Are you confused? Don't know what to do? I was too, but it's not the end. If I could regain my health, then so can you. Do you want to know how? Just keep reading and you will find tips that can help you overcome, step by step, this difficult stage of your life. You will also find some tips that will be useful in the event that you contract COVID-19, since I also suffered from this disease.

# Confusion

The hardest time of my life was when I was informed that I had been infected with HPV. Two months after the birth of my son I began to feel pain in my lower belly and experience unusual bleeding. I made an appointment with a gynecologist to look for a diagnosis and as a prevention she ordered some tests to detect HPV, she informed me that the results would arrive between three and seven days. When you are in a state of anxiety and want to know what is going on, the wait becomes eternal. Three days passed and I did not get any answer, at that time I was very anxious, the minutes seemed like hours and the hours days. I am convinced that, like me, many women go through the same situation of frustration and anxiety about waiting. After a few more days I received the call from the gynecologist with a disastrous news: I had HPV in stage 16, my world collapsed, and that's when I panicked; confusion, fear, despair, shame and guilt ensued.

I had a terrible confusion because I didn't know what I should do, I wasn't properly informed about the virus and I didn't really understand what that virus consists of and what you can do.

I was afraid of not knowing what would happen to my body from that moment on.

I felt desperate to want to fix the problem instantly.

I felt embarrassed as I thought I was the only woman in the world with HPV without counting that some gynecologists aren't professional and make you feel worse. If you are in a situation like this, with HPV, I recommend that you go to your medical consultations accompanied by a friend, with your mother, your husband, someone who will give you the moral support you need and so you will not feel so alone and embarrassed in this situation.

The feeling of guilt I think is the strongest. I felt that it was all my fault for being with the wrong person at the wrong time, you feel that it is your fault what is happening to you and since it is your fault you deserve to be sick. The reality is that all these feelings together are only a fig of your imagination and only make you feel more pain and see more things in your body than there really are. The gynecologist told me that HPV does not cause symptoms and that many people live with the virus and sometimes don't even realize what they have, I know we are all different.

However, I think something changes in your body, even if it is something insignificant, such as vaginal discharge, presence of itching, burning, unusual bleeding, even low back pain. From my personal point of view, I do not believe that a virus, especially if it is high risk, which sometimes has serious consequences on your body, will not give you signs of its presence. We should be on the lookout for any abnormal changes in our body and have routine body checkups regularly.

But now what? That is the question that we all ask ourselves and that doctors answer half-heartedly, they do not explain the information, they only tell you that you should continue with your routine checkups and wait to see what will happen in your body, they leave you without a very wide range of information: it can become a cancer or be nothing.

Hearing the word cancer is terrifying, I could not believe that this was happening to me, I was always a monogamous woman, but my husband did have relations with another person and a few days after that I began to experience excessive vaginal discharge, I was very scared and that was when I found out what happened, when I was pregnant with eight months of gestation, I went to the nearest emergency room and there I explained my situation, they ordered to do some studies of sexually transmitted diseases, but for some reason nobody ordered to do the HPV test, I only received some antibiotics and an injection, when the results arrived everything was fine and at that time I still did not have a maternity doctor assigned since I had moved from another city. When I found a doctor, I explained my situation again and he decided that I should continue with the antibiotics, but he did not order the HPV test either.

I knew that virus existed, but I wasn't informed enough of what it was and the consequences that catching it could have, so I was more worried about not having other diseases that you normally hear about or talk about more. HPV is one of the sexually transmitted diseases that is not talked about much and there is not much information about it, from the point of view of medicine. I was worried about chlamydia, gonorrhea,

HIV; none of this came out positive or on the two occasions in which I did the examinations as I thought that everything was alright, I thought that it was a contamination by fungi or bacteria what was causing the vaginal discharge.

When the day of giving birth came, the doctor continued with the antibiotics to make sure my baby was okay, everything happened normally and, calmly, I returned home after two days. However, I continued with the symptoms of pain of lower belly and lower back and a little vaginal discharge, I thought it was a result of childbirth, but time was passing, and the symptoms were getting worse, so, in my opinion, I think that when you get the virus something changes in your body, only that people sometimes do not realize, not because there are no changes, but because they do not pay enough attention to their bodies.

Viruses are microorganisms composed of genetic material protected by a protein envelope that causes various diseases, introducing themselves as a parasite (yes, you read correctly, a parasite) into a cell to replicate in it since these do not replicate on their own. There are two types of viruses, DNA and RNA. The papillomavirus is of the DNA type, which needs an epithelium for its replication and thus completes its life cycle. When the virus is already in your body, in your cells there are three problems that the virus causes in order to make more copies of itself:

1. How to reproduce inside the infected cell?
2. How to spread from one host to another?
3. How to avoid being eliminated by the defenses of the immune system?

Yes, the virus looks for ways to avoid being eliminated by your immune system. HPV is transmitted sexually, therefore, it is preventable and can be curable, but not having much information about this you live in great confusion, as I was, I think a big concern is to think if you will really live with HPV for the rest of your life as you are led to believe, so it is important to clarify that each organism fights the virus for which it has been infected. The cells of the immune system of each infected person will fight this virus and the better the state of your immune system, the greater the tools it will have to fight the virus with antibodies. In the following chapters you will learn how to boost your immune system and how to deal with the virus from an emotional point of view, since contracting the virus is devastating, I can't speak for men, but I think it affects them emotionally as well. I know that if you are a woman and you get the virus it is exhausting because it touches every aspect of your life, the relationship with your partner. the relationship with your family and the relationship with yourself, the mental part, the spiritual part and, of course, the physical part, but you are not the only one, there are millions of cases like yours and mine, for this reason I am sharing my experience, I want you to know that you are not alone and I want to give you a little support and hope in these difficult times.

# What you need to know

This chapter is one of the most important in this book. Right now, you're probably looking for information to get rid of HPV. I spent tons of money and time on taking medication I didn't need. There were also many things I couldn't find. I advise you not to jump from one product to another indiscriminately trying to heal yourself. Start with a medicine that seems right to you and give it time to see if it works.

I know that there are many people selling hope and that, precisely, is my purpose with this book. I want to help you help yourself. The best advice I can give to overcome HPV, or any disease is to start with your diet. It is a proven fact that your body heals itself. What you introduce into your body as food can help or harm that process. Some examples are smoking and drinking, that, mixed with poor diet will not provide any solution. I consumed meats all my life, as well as sugar, but when I had to choose between my health or junk food, without hesitation I chose my health. It is not easy to achieve, since it is very rooted habit, but over time we can all adapt to anything. I followed a vegan diet for a couple of years and found products with which I could substitute meats and sugars. I will guide you as you read the nutritional chapter. My intention with this book is to explain HPV since the Internet does not have enough information about all the possible variants of this disease, in my case not even the doctor warned me or advised me about my life expectancy when I got HPV. There are many types of HPV, some of those listed as high-risk are known as 16 and 18, but publicly available information only mentions those that are more common.

Since this disease becomes many types of cancers, it is responsible for 80% of cancerous lesions of the cervix and other types of cancers such as cancer of the anus, vulva, vagina, penis, also throat cancer and, in some cases, even head cancer. Other complications that appear with these types of viruses are flat warts, which although no one tells you about it, exist and they come out on your hands, soles of the feet and in your throat if you are infected with the virus in that area, but there are more than two hundred types of HPV classified as high risk such as those I already mentioned and there are also low risk, which are 6, 11, 30, 44 among many others, these are the causes of genital warts. They also manifest themselves in different parts of the body such as the hands and soles of the feet. Sometimes doctors, even on the Internet, may tell you that some of these kinds of viruses don't have any symptoms. But one of the other symptoms, which in my personal experience I noticed, was a stabbing pain in my left ear, although this can occur in either of your ears. If you observe this symptom, the recommendation I can give you is to boil the water equivalent to a cup with a piece of fresh ginger for five minutes, let it cool and place a few drops in your ears. Another thing you can use is warm towels, this will soothe the pain. A symptom that usually occurs is dry and scratchy throat, however, once these symptoms have manifested it is very likely that it has spread to your mouth and throat. There are many types of oils that I will list in the supplements (healing foods) chapter to help you overcome the disease. Another tip I can offer you to improve your throat symptoms is to stop oral sex, just until the HPV symptoms go away, especially if your throat is still normal. Other information I got is that it takes many years for cancer to develop from HPV, in my experience I developed precancer about a year I was infected. After 10 years have elapsed, this information will no longer be valid. It might be better to say: "in my experience I developed precancer a year after I was infected". But I'm not sure if it was.

One symptom that I began to experience was pain in my right leg. Sometimes, when you have cancer or precancer in some of your organs, other organs react. Other conditions may result in epithelial lesions, these are abnormal cells that form on the surface of certain organs, such as the cervix, vagina, vulva and anus. With CIN1 (stage 1 cervical intraepithelial neoplasia) in my cervix, which quickly became CIN 2 and then CIN 3 after three months. In my case, I suffered from this condition in my vagina, I did not know that I could develop this sickness, and no one told me that it existed until I began to feel a slight stabbing pain right in the vaginal labia. When I observed I realized that my skin was changing, some parts of my skin were very red and with the passage of the days they were becoming black and transformed to the white color. At this point the skin of that area looked very white, it seems that it had fish scales, there are two ways to treat this condition from the point of view of medicine: if it is already a very advanced lesion, like the one I have, your gynecologist can remove it they can using a technique called cryotherapy which basically consists of freezing your cells so that they do not become a cancer. All these changes can be prevented since they are your cells that can become a cancer, as I already mentioned.

In the chapter on genital care for men and women you will find information to prevent or prevent the return of the lesion. Know that when you suffer from HPV it increases by up to 50% the risk of contracting other sexually transmitted diseases, such as HIV, chlamydia, gonorrhea, among many others. Some of these diseases cannot be prevented using only condoms since they are highly contagious as is HPV that is transmitted only with genital contact, so it is important to reduce the number of sexual partners or, as a more definite measure, practice abstinence which is the most effective way to prevent and not spread sexual health diseases.

As I mentioned earlier, I contracted HPV while pregnant and one of my big concerns was whether my son might have been infected with the virus. I also worried about what would happen if I had it and what consequences could be brought, so I scheduled an appointment with a pediatrician, she explained that there was a high risk that my baby could have a condition called RRP, for having been a vaginal birth and for having breastfed my son for three months, since in this way the virus is treated from mother to child. RRP stands for a disease called recurrent respiratory papillomatosis or laryngeal papillomatosis, tumors called papilloma's that grow in the airways that run from the nose and mouth to the lungs (the so-called respiratory tract). Although tumors can grow anywhere in the respiratory tract, they most commonly develop in the larynx, which is called laryngeal papillomatosis. Papilloma's can vary in size and grow very quickly; they often grow back after they have been removed. This is a serious condition that can cause serious health problems in children, even in adults it can cause voice changes or a harsh or hoarse voice when PRR papilloma's interfere with normal vibrations of the vocal cords, eventually PRR tumors can block the passage of air into the airways and cause difficulty breathing. The symptoms of PRR tend to be more severe in children as they may have difficulty breathing when sleeping or may have difficulty swallowing and other conditions such as asthma or chronic bronchitis and in some cases the severity of the case can lead to death.

It is said that, usually, the viruses that cause this condition are low-risk and in very rare cases high-risk. From my personal experience I can affirm that high-risk viruses also cause this clinical picture, generating flat warts and tumors in your throat, in men, women and children with HPV.

# What you should do

If you are ready to fight the virus, start here.

A good tip that I can give you before starting do not obsess about things, because you eat large amounts of vegetables, fruits or supplements at once doesn't mean you will get rid of the disease. The virus, as I mentioned above, begins to be fought with dietary changes, but you must do it with moderation, perseverance and with a lot of patience.

The first thing you should do is start detoxifying your body, the detoxication is in fact, the most important part of the process because we will eliminate the toxins that, in most cases, alter health and weaken your immune system. With a weakened immune system, it will be impossible to get rid of the virus.

How to detoxify your body? How many ways you do it? You can use herbs in the form of tea such as dandelion, this plant helps you eliminate retained fluids and purify the blood, fighting bacteria, in addition to being rich in vitamin A, folic acid and fiber.

Red clover helps eliminate toxins from your body, it also stimulates the production of bile helping to improve digestion, you can alternate between teas and apple cider vinegar since this is also a good detoxifier and is rich in vitamins A and B. The way you can prepare it is to add a tablespoon of apple cider vinegar in a glass of water, just like teas. This should be taken in the mornings, at least for fifteen days. In this period in which you are detoxifying your body. You must begin to change your eating style, do not think that because you begin to make a strict diet which makes you of hunger, there are different ways to stay healthy, fight the virus and at the same time is not hungry, but obviously to change your way of feeding step by step. You cannot do it from one day to another because your body is exposed to a *shock* and you would begin to feel dizziness, tiredness and headaches. It matters that when you have already changed your diet you stand firm. It is difficult at the beginning, but it is not impossible. Being constant to obtain results in a short period of time. Try to start eliminating all meat! Also eliminate pasta, rice (brown and white), bread, potatoes, starch or corn, tortillas, cereal, cookies, fried foods, etc. All these foods are cooked with sugar in your body a few minutes after having ingested them. Eliminate all kinds of drinks such as juices with artificial color, sodas and energy drinks, these products contain large amounts of refined sugar which is one of the most important things that you must eliminate from your diet. This is very harmful to your health and at the same time strengthens the HPV in your body for a period of in definite time. You should not consume any canned products, as they contain a dangerous chemical called bisphenol A.

You should stop consuming milk and all milk products, such as cheese, yogurt, ice cream, among others. Milk contains harmful bacteria that cause inflammation in your organs and, over time. You will be prone to suffer from multiple osteoporosis and allergies. It is also highly recommended to eliminate all soy products, since, in the long term, it can cause different cancers such as breast and uterus, among other diseases.

You should also eliminate canola and corn oils as they are harmful to your health. In the chapter dedicated to foods that heal you will find a wide variety of natural oils for cooking that are very healthy.

You should focus, as much as possible, on living a life without being stress, this is very important. I know that sometimes it is very difficult, almost impossible. I was in this very situation, however, to stay strong, not to suffer from stress is important to be able to continue fighting against HPV. This is a bad ally that, over time, becomes a powerful enemy as it can worsen your immune or physical health. If stress remains present you will be accompanied by HPV for longer.

You should cultivate the habit of sleeping and rest well because whenever you sleep your body releases hormones that help fight diseases. These hormones called melanin and serotonin also help to control the effects of the stress hormone. The suggestion is to sleep, at least, eight hours a day.

Being in a situation like this requires a high dose of patience, having the HPV leaves you desperate, you just want to solve that problem quickly, you want to find all the things that can help you at the right time, but unfortunately it is not so. It requires great patience to continue fighting correctly, impatience makes you do wrong things and make many mistakes that lead you down a longer path.

Another thing you should do is monitor and control your PH. Having a balanced pH is essential to be able to get rid of the virus and other diseases so you must maintain a pH above 7, that is, at an alkaline level. An alkaline pH is the best guarantee of health, the cells of the body need a slightly alkaline pH – between 7 and 7.4 – to function properly because an organism with an acidic pH is a breeding ground for many diseases. The causes of an imbalanced pH and an acidic body are an unbalanced diet and poor nutrition.

Heating food in the microwave is very harmful to your health, as well as bad habits such as smoking and drinking alcohol, stress, lack of exercise, consumption of products high in sugar and highly refined and processed products such as table salt, and foods that have added these refined products such as peanuts, pistachios, coffee, etc.

An excellent recommendation to keep your body alkalized more quickly is to drink water with lemon, it is recommended to drink warm water in the morning with a lemon, since this is the most alkalizing fruit on the planet, in addition to being rich in vitamin C and also helps fight cancer, as well as it is a good aid in beautiful skin because it helps stop the appearance of wrinkles. The method to measure your pH: just put a container with the second urine of the morning – the first is very acidic – and immerse in it a tip of the pH indicator. You can find these indicators in any pharmacy and amazon. Now that you know what to do, let's move on to the best part, the foods that heal!

# Foods that heal

HPV is a resistant virus, but if you do not fight it it will stay in your body and wreak havoc that can be irreversible in some cases, it is important that you consume the foods that heal. It all starts with your eating style, so let's get started! I know sometimes it's hard to find all the supplements, but I can help you.

Fruits and vegetables are very easy to get and it is very important that you incorporate them into your new lifestyle. Basically, you will eat a diet based on nuts, vegetables and fresh fruits. You can also incorporate healthy flours such as spelt flour and semolina, you can find a wide variety of products derived from spelt and semolina such as bread and pasta and you can even make your own recipes with these raw materials such as pancakes, tortillas and many other things. You will find these recipes in the book "Recipes to Combat HPV".

Other supplements that help a lot are natural oils, you can consume them incorporated into your tea and some others that you can use to cook. Oregano oil is a powerful antiviral, antibacterial and antifungal, you can put three drops of oregano oil in a cup of tea. Oregano tea is very easy to get, as it is available in almost all supermarkets.

Tea tree oil is excellent for fighting bacteria. Almond oil is a rich source of vitamin E. Blackseed oil is a powerful anti-inflammatory and antibacterial, muscle soothing and antioxidant, among many other benefits. Star anise oil is used to cure menstrual cramps, plus it is antiseptic and antioxidant. The ideal oils for cooking and that provide a wide variety of vitamins and help strengthen your immune system are avocado oil since it is rich in omega 3, vitamins and contains many antioxidants. It is excellent for cooking, as well as grape seed oil that is rich in vitamins C and K and has a large amount of vitamin E, helps against inflammations and strengthens your immune system. Coconut oil is natural and is an excellent ally to fight the virus as it helps to reduce inflammation of the organs, is rich in vitamin E, in addition to helping to fight the fungus called *Candida albicans*.

Vitamin B12, vitamin D, like vitamin E, can be found in pill form, but at the same time you can get them by consuming fruits and vegetables. Supplements such as ginger pills, evening primrose seed oil, flax*seed* oil, zinc, spirulina, magnesium, are excellent options.

Red fruits are magnificent because they are rich in vitamins and antioxidant is, among them are strawberries, pomegranates, blackberries, cherries, blueberries, plums, grapes, cranberry (lingonberry), watermelon and others. There are fruits whose consumption is also very important for their high content of vitamins such as papaya, oranges, pina, grapefruit, bananas, pears, peaches, kiwi, figs, mandarins, apples, melon, dragon fruit, lichee (fruit of

Chinese origin), persimmon or rosewood, mangoes, guava, mangosteen. A fruit that is always good for your diet is soursop, known as Gaviola in Mexico. This fruit has great health benefits because it is hydrating, rich in vitamins and minerals, decreases arterial tension thanks to its high potassium content. It relieves anemia because it has a high iron content, it is a good ally against osteoporosis, it is rich in calcium and phosphorous. It has a high antioxidant power thanks to its high content of vitamin C that helps us against the oxidation of cells. Soursop extract reduces the progression of tumors in cancer. This wonderful food can be found in the form of fruit, tea or powder to make smoothies and natural capsules. Make sure be careful with the seeds, if you are going to consume the soursop in its fruit form you must remove all the seeds because they can be toxic. Other fruits rich in vitamins are durian, jackfruit, avocado and tamarind. The black elderberry is another important fruit to consume because it is rich in antioxidant and vitamins that help strengthen your immune system. It also helps with inflammation processes, with stress and cold symptoms, in addition to protecting your heart and it is a powerful anticancer. You must also consume a large amount of chlorophyll daily to strengthen your immune system, in addition chlorophyll eliminates the fungi in your body, detoxifies your blood, cleanses your intestines, prevents the cancer and provides energy to and at the same time to alkalize your body and balances your pH becoming a less conducive environment for bacteria to grow and cause different diseases. Chlorophyll can be found in green vegetables such as: chard, spinach, romaine lettuce, endives, chicory, okra, cactus, celery, bell green, coriander, parsley, green tomatoes, aloe vera, jalapeno, squash, broccoli, bitter melon, brussels sprouts, asparagus, rucola, cucumber, zucchini. Kale is among the most nutrient-dense foods on the planet, it has a lot of chlorophyll. It works as an anti-inflammatory, provides antioxidant, calcium, and potassium. It is rich in vitamins A, C, E and K. You can prepare in salads or smoothies with a fruit of your preference.

Other plant elements that help a lot with your immune system are herbs consumed in infusions or as tea. A powerful plant called *Gynostema pentaphyllum* or jiaogulan, taken as an infusion, helps you fight HPV. It fights all kinds of viruses, in addition to helping to fight asthma, migraines and chronic bronchitis; it protects cells against oxidation and is a powerful antioxidant. Oregano tea like oregano oil is antiviral, antifungal and antibacterial, if you combine the tea with three drops of oil it is double the effect. Damiana tea (or tea from Mexico) helps you fight the virus and clean your reproductive system and if you already suffer from cervical dysplasia it is important that you start consuming it. Green tea helps you boost your immune system and helps fight cancer; this tea is a powerful antioxidant that helps with cell regeneration. Star anise tea helps you regulate your menstrual period and is antispasmodic. You can combine the tea with a few drops of the essential oil obtained from this plant. Mangosteen tea is wonderful for its large number of properties. It helps strengthen your immune system; it is an antioxidant that controls blood sugar. It also helps with urinary tract infections and is used to treat gonorrhea, fungal infections in the mouth, tuberculosis and irregular menstrual periods. Nettle tea is rich in vitamins A, C and K, in addition to its power to detoxify, it is expectorant and antiallergic. Rosemary tea is an excellent natural antibiotic, anti-inflammatory, plus it helps with stress and for women who are already in menopause, or premenopausal. It helps to calm the symptoms. Calendula tea or other calendula products, such as oil, or calendula ointments work as antifungals, regulates your menstrual periods, it is an antiseptic, helps with burns and bumps, also helps fight dermatitis and even to reduce fever you can consume it in different ways. You can even eat its petals in salads or use it as an enema, if you are infected with HPV in that area it will be of great help to reduce genital warts and helps with hemorrhoids. Dandelion tea helps fight viral infections, helps with fluid retention and in turn detoxifies the blood. Ginger tea is good for fighting all kinds of viruses, combined with lemon brings many benefits to your health, in addition to stimulating your metabolism to make weight loss easier. Echinacea tea boosts your immune system, relieves sore throats and is effective against the flu. Another herb that you can consume in the form of tea and helps a lot to eliminate HPV is cat's claw, as it is a powerful antioxidant, anti-inflammatory, strengthens the immune system and helps fight genital herpes.

Remember that you cannot use refined sugar of any kind to sweeten the tea, but you can replace it with agave syrup since it is a powerful sweetener, this is extracted from a plant like a cactus, but that really is from the family of the aloe vera and is 100% natural, also has anti-inflammatory properties, antibacterial as well as strengthens your immune system and is ideal for diabetic people, as it helps regulate blood sugar. Another natural sweetener you can use is honey, but this must be honey raw natural honey. Another powerful ally to fight against the virus is black garlic since it is antiviral, antimicrobial, improves your immune system, prevents migraines and helps fight some types of cancer, you can consume it naturally or in the form of capsules.

It is important to consume foods rich in proteins, however, they must be foods that provide proteins of vegetable origin since you cannot consume protein of animals. You can find the protein in amaranth since it is a superfood that contains, iron, Phosphorus, vitamins, A, B, C and D among many others. Chickpeas have the most vegetable protein, decreases cholesterol, has a high content of fiber, contains omega 6, antioxidant is like zinc and selenium, it is important to the improvement of the skin and the digestion.

Quinoa is another protein-rich food, it has up to 23% more protein than many other foods. Consuming quinoa helps prevent colon cancer and other diseases as it has a lot of vitamins, phosphorus, omega 6, antioxidants and is delicious. Consuming lentils regularly will provide you with a small amount of protein and fiber, in addition to helping to prevent anemia due to its large amount of iron. Wild rice is a wonderfully balanced food source, providing a healthy blend of protein and fiber, containing antioxidant elements is and plays a role in maintaining the health of your cells.

Coconut milk has protein, it is anti-inflammatory, prevents anemia, ulcers and blood sugar. Chía seeds have a high proportion of protein, help control hunger, are a great source of omega 3. Flaxseeds are rich in proteins, fibers, vitamins, prevent certain types of cancer and help reduce stress.

Consuming all these foods and natural supplements will help you keep your immune system strengthened so your body won't be stuck with HPV.

# Genital care for men and women

It is important that I mention genital care in men since there is not much talk of HPV when it comes to men. Most of the time, men are carriers of the virus and if they do not realize that they have it there is a possibility that, over time, they will develop penis cancer, throat cancer, as well as anus cancer, especially if you are one of the LGBT community. You must take good care your genital area and do everything possible to stop the virus, all the natural remedies indicated here can be done by both men and women, because in women it can prevent a cervical dysplasia or epithelial lesions in the genital area. And in Man and Women with HPV You will suffer from genital warts in this way, we will control their growth and eliminate those that already exist. How will we do this? With herbs and natural oils.

How to prepare the first remedy:

**Ingredients:**

- 6 cloves of garlic (average estimated amount)
- Tea tree oil

**Preparation:**

The amount of garlic will depend on how extensive the affected area is, you can add or remove. You must mash the garlic very well to form a paste, put fifteen drops of tea tree and mix both ingredients well. Then you must spread that paste on the affected area and cover it with a band aid. It is advisable to spread petroleum jelly around the area where you applied the garlic paste and oil, so that mixture does not touch the area that is not affected by warts. We must remember that garlic is very strong and can burn your skin if you are not careful. If you apply it every day the warts are going to burn little by little. You must apply the paste and leave it overnight, then in the next morning you remove it with enough water. To achieve a better effectiveness, you can remove the garlic paste with rosemary tea this plant contains elements that work as a powerful natural antibiotic and you can find it dry or fresh in any supermarket. For the preparation of rosemary tea need 114 g (4 ounces) of rosemary per liter of water, boil for ten minutes, remove from heat and let cool to room temperature. With this preparation you can wash your genital area very well.

## Genital washes

It is important that genital washes are not done daily because, although we will only use natural products, these can also change the pH of your genital area from alkaline to acid and what we want is to maintain an alkaline pH since this will be easier to fight the virus but remember that everything in excess can be counterproductive. It is important that, for any washing you do with the plants suggested here, you remove all excess from the plant until there is only the liquid left to perform the washes. This can be easily done with a strainer or a fabric sieve.

## Vaginal washing with arnica

This is a very easy plant to get, the arnica washes are very efficient because it can end up with discomfort such as itching or burning. Arnica has antiseptic properties the arnica is a very effective healing for open wounds. If you have a dysplasia cervical the application of arnica is highly recommended because this will prevent the appearance of new infections and at the same time help you to regenerate the cells of your Cervix

## Vaginal washes with calendula

Calendula is another plant whose components have great antibiotic properties that you can use for washing. Its use can prevent and help healing as it is antibacterial. Genital washes should be performed with two tablespoons of calendula for each liter of water, you could also exchange between vaginal washes of one plant or another every third day.

### Pennyroyal washes

Pennyroyal is a plant whose properties serve as antifungal, antibacterial and anti-inflammatory. You must use 30 g of pennyroyal for each liter of water, put on the fire and let it boil for at least ten minutes and then let stand for thirty minutes or until it is at room temperature.

### Washes with heather or basil

Basil is another powerful plant with many natural anti-septic and sedative properties that, in addition to helping with the HPV virus, also helps fight urinary infections and it has sedative properties will favor of pain in your genital area. Two tablespoons of basil leaves should be boiled for five minutes in half a liter of water, when it is at room temperature remove the excess of the plant and perform vaginal washing with the remaining liquid. (This infusion should not be ingested).

### Witch- hazel washes

Witch- hazel, also known as hazel, is a plant with very prominent anti-inflammatory properties, helps treat circulation and hemorrhoids and is ideal if you suffer from an epithelial injury or to prevent it. You must add three tablespoons for each liter of water and boil for ten minutes, when the water has settled and is at room temperature, remove the excess and wash.

### Chamomile washes

Another plant that you can use to do vaginal washes is chamomile since it has soothing and antimicrobial properties and can be used as a vaginal douche. You should add four tablespoons of chamomile per half liter of water and boil for five minutes. The application is similar to the previous ones.

### Washed with malva

Malva is a medicinal plant that possesses antiseptic, anti-inflammatory and antifungal properties. Three tablespoons of mauve should be added for each liter of water, boiled for ten minutes and add five drops of tea tree oil, after cooling use as a vaginal wash.

### OVULES of natural products

Another product you can use is vaginal ovules made with natural products. These ovules can also be used by men, in their rectal area or simply applied to the penis and the entire genital area. Ovules, in conjunction with vaginal washes, are effective in eliminating the virus in the genital area and avoid other complications.

### Aloe ovules

Aloe vera is a good ally for the defenses since it helps eliminate dead cells, is healing and a powerful natural anti-inflammatory. Its antioxidant properties are perfect for reducing inflammation and it is rich in vitamins and minerals. Preparation mode: cut the aloe vera by removing all the skin from the bark very well until only the inner part that is semi-transparent remains, wash very well with cold water and store in the fridge. Aloe crystals cut into small pieces can be used throughout the night and make sure to expel them the next morning.

## Capsules with coconut oil

Ovules with coconut oil have vitamins E and K, a combination of ideal ingredients that moisturize skin tissues and strengthen cell regeneration. This in turn boosts your immune system. You should prepare 227 g (8 ounces) of coconut oil combination with ten drops of oil of tree oil since this oil is antibacterial and antifungal. It is important to know that you should never ingest the oil tea tree because it is harmful or when use orally. It is also important to use the correct dose for vaginal Washes, you should not put too much oil as it can cause irritation or dryness of the skin. Coconut oil should mix very well with the oil of tree oil, put in clean recipient covered and put in the fridge for at least three hours. It should use of daily application.

## Rosemary Ovules

Another plant you can use to make eggs is rosemary. It is preferable that you use fresh rosemary, so you take advantage of all its properties since there are many, it is a powerful antispasmodic, antibacterial and antiseptic, among many other properties. For its preparation you should put 227 g (8 ounces) of rosemary in a glass refractory and cover it with almond oil. This oil is anti-inflammatory and rich in vitamin E, you should let it rest for at least a month in a dark place. After that time, you should put it in the fridge and use it as eggs or simply rub on the affected areas.

## Garlic and coconut oil Ovules

You can also use garlic as it is a natural antibiotic and antifungal, making it ideal for fighting HPV and many other kinds of viral diseases. It has a high antioxidant power and is rich in vitamins C and B6, in its composition healthy minerals such as calcium and manganese are also present. To prepare the Ovules you must use a few cloves of garlic and organic coconut oil (100% natural) with a few drops of essential oil from tree oil. Cut the garlic or mush to form a paste place it in a container and cover it with a tablespoon of coconut oil, a tablespoon of oil tree tea and a tablespoon of grapeseed oil. Let that preparation sit in the fridge for a week. At the end of that time, you can use it by applying it as a daily ovule. You can also use natural garlic as a vaginal ovule, remove the skin from the garlic, use it with gauze and tie it to a thread to ensure that it does not stay inside the vagina.

All applications of vaginal ovules are preferred to perform at night, as well as these act during the sleep period. Vaginal washing can be done at any time of the day, but it is recommended that you do them before going to sleep, so that after the vaginal washing you can use the ovules to get better results. It is important to remember that when preparing eggs or vaginal washes try to use organic products and sterilize all the containers that you are going to use and do it moderately and with caution since the genital area is a delicate area. Genital care is of vital importance to prevent the appearance of infections and eliminate HPV.

# Don't despair

Feeling that you no longer have hope to get out of this health problem such as HPV can cause a depressive crisis, and when you are immersed in depression, the only thing that can get you out of that dead end is hope, but it is so difficult to have hope in that situation.

Sometimes you feel like you're running out of strength and you just want to stop everything, go back to your normal life and forget that you have the virus. It is strenuous to be attending gynecological appointments; doing strict diets; live in fear of what will happen in the coming months; feel that no one cares, since everyone continues with the normal course of their vines, but no one really stops to ask you what you really feel or need; no one tries to understand you.

In my personal situation I came to be with severe depression, to this day I am struggling to get to have a normal life again. The experience of living with HPV and ending up with a cancer was traumatic and depressing for me. Spending days in bed with high fevers, I just wanted to disappear. I cried whole nights I felt absolutely miserable, not important, guilty and empty. The fact that all this happened in the period of my pregnancy and when I gave birth, I think I already felt depressed. Living through all this was comparable to living a nightmare, I felt so tired, I couldn't focus on anything. I could not sleep, I lost my appetite, I weighed only 98pounds! I was in really bad condition, I had a great lack of self-esteem, I felt that I was nobody, taking antidepressants and consulting a psychologist. Fortunately, I was able to find a website called Better Help that wasn't that expensive. If you don't have a medical study, the costs for treatments can be expensive.

Every country is different, but I think in all of them you can locate resources that can help you. If you are feeling some of the symptoms or emotions described in this book, I recommend that you fight not to go to extremes because then it will be more difficult to recover your health, both bodily and mental. If you are a woman and you are depressed and experiencing those feelings of emptiness and lack of self-esteem, I recommend that you have spent something for you every day; How to fix your hair or make up, even if you are at home; walking or doing some outdoor activity for at least 30 minutes. I suggest you do \ this for yourself, for your mental health. Writing is also an excellent therapy, write down everything you feel.

Here I teach you a psychotherapy exercise to help you discover new ways of thinking, behaving, and find ways to change habits that contribute to depression getting worse. Make a table in a notebook, discover five of your qualities, those that make you unique. Find out, for example, what you like about your appearance.

I also suggest you do tasks that you did before, even if it is something small or, such as checking mail, folding clothes, anything; this will help you not to feel useless.

**Breathing exercise**

I also offer you a relaxation exercise that I suggest you do, it is excellent for relaxing and being able to sleep, it will provide you with mental clarity and will lead you to a state of inner peace. Find a quiet place, sit in a comfortable position, with your eyes closed. You will perform conscious breathing, be sure to inhale through your nose and exhale through your mouth. Slow down the rhythm of your breathing, counting slowly as you inhale and exhale and performing this process in a gentle and relaxed way. Try to hold your breath for a second or two, then exhale slowly through your mouth. I suggest you do this for at least five minutes, twice a day. You can start when you are not anxious or stressed, with the practice these simple exercises will help you to have self-control of your emotions.

A good recommendation I can give you is to drink lemonade. It has glucose, in simple terms, glucose is fuel for the brain. Acts of self-control reduce blood glucose levels. Willpower can be restored by raising the level of good blood sugar in your blood, so drink a glass of agave-sweetened lemonade to strengthen your ability to stay in control, since the power you may have over your emotions will help you develop your inner strength and be able to guide you through the hardest situations of your life, resisting adversity and thus be able to emerge stronger from the most complicated circumstances. It is important to have the support and or of other people, but the most important thing is that you find your own inner strength to move forward and not give up. Not giving up depends on you, so begin to forgive yourself, learn to relax, to see or read something motivating and remember every day that you are a valuable person.

# The Fears

It has been a great challenge for me to write this book, but at the same time it has been a way to try to heal inwardly. I have left a little my fears, frustration and sadness. I shed a few tears writing, but I think in the end it was worth the effort because I feel more liberated from my emotions. It has been a long and traumatic journey, I have not overcome everything, since somewhere in me, there is a bit of trauma that makes me feel insecure and afraid, it is the type of fear that does not allow me to trust anyone.

Having HPV or precancer – especially the word cancer – makes you feel close to death and makes you see life from another perspective, that feeling is traumatizing, not to mention that when I was going through those difficult moments COVID-19 appeared.

I contracted papillomavirus and pneumonia at the same time, those were the days when I wondered why me? I blamed God for everything. But I believe that in the end God has a purpose for everyone because, despite all the difficulties, I am still here.

When I came out positive for COVID-19 I started doing everything I did before, but in duplicate. Now I had a smoothie nine times a day, I found a powerful plant called eucalyptus with which I prepared a magnificent tea, which is used to combat respiratory problems, has decongestant action, promotes inflammation of the airways, relieves cough and symptoms of COVID-19. You can use it as a tea and use it in hot water and alcohol baths. COVID-19 is just another virus that pierces your immune system, so I was desperately trying to strengthen my immune system, as I was receiving chemotherapy at the time.

Another excellent tea that helped me a lot with the strengthening of my immune system was Reishi mushroom tea or also known as *Ganoderma lucidum* or Lingzhi, it is a mushroom native to Asia, but you can also find it in America. it is obtained fresh, in the form of tea, in capsules, in pills or in powder, if you find it in powder you can add it to your smoothies to change the flavor. This fungus keeps your immune system high, therefore, it makes it easier for the body to have defense against any disease. Vitamins, antioxidants, and most importantly, helps the regeneration of your cells, for that reason orals protects you from HPV. It also helps in repairing tissues in all parts of your body. Vitamin C has many antioxidants, antioxidants are nourishing that provide a blockage for your skin and your cells against free radiation which occurs when your body decomposes food or when it is exposed to tobacco smoke or, as in my case, that was exposed to radiation or chemotherapy.

I have learned a lot during these last years, it is sad to think that only when extreme things happen to you is when the meaning of your life changes, you positively change your eating habits, as well as you learn to take care of yourself and those around you. If you are reading this book, I recommend that you try to follow all my advice so that you do not reach the health condition in which I find myself. If I would have had a book like this in my hands from the beginning of the HPV process, I know that my life would have been different.

It took me a lot of time and effort, especially the time, to try every product I found and wait to see the reactions that were occurring in my body. All this that is written here was tested by me and were the products with los that I was getting better. I know that each person is different, therefore, each organism is different, but the viruses are the same, the viruses of to the risk are all the same, the virus of low risk are all the same, what differentiates them is that they are composed of different microorganisms, but they are viruses in the end.

Another important aspect is how your body reacts when it goes from the acidic condition to the alkaline condition. No virus, whether high or low risk, can survive in an alkaline environment, what kills the virus in one person kills it in another because they are composed of the same thing, how fast will it do it? It depends on your organism. It take about three years to learn all this, as I said before, no one explains what HPV is and what it can really cause, in addition to cancer or the erroneous. I had papilloma's in my throat, I underwent an operation to remove them. My throat had an invasion of cells called hyperplasia which is the first stated the cancer. Have another condition medical term called intraductal

Papilloma's of the breasts. There are papilloma's or warts in the milk ducts of the breasts that caused me a lot of pain, in addition to producing the secretion of a thick fluid of yellowish color and bad smell. These papilloma's spread quick and I had to undergo another surgery to remove them since this is the only possibility to take them out. Another part of my body that came out or infected with papilloma's was the colon. These cause a lot of pain, itching and sometimes even bleeding, it is uncomfortable and painful. I have not undergone any surgery since I am trying to eradicate them naturally by making enemas of calendula and using lime ointment marigold, also applying baths with the grass called Cat Claw and arnica, since the cat claws destroys the papillomavirus.

I am also consuming many cherries, as these are rich in vitamins A, D and E, folic acid, beta-carotene and have a high fiber content. The fiber helps the correct digestion, the intense red color of the fruit is contributed by the large amount of antioxidants that it has, among which the Quercetina, the Lutein and the Zeaxanthin stand out, also it provides minerals such as magnesium, iron and calcium. And something additional: it helps you sleep better since it contains melatonin.

Making use of all these products and always focusing on the organic and the natural, I have been able to observe an improvement, they no longer bleed as much, and the inflammation was reduced. The colonoscopy showed 20% less papilloma's in the Pap smear exam, the HPV disappeared meaning that everything I'm doing is helping to reduce the number of papilloma's and eliminate HPV.

However, the positive results from the use of natural and organic products were not only limited to HPV, but also helped me with the COVID-19 virus and the pneumonia, since I was only two weeks with the virus.

So, as you can see, I have had a traumatic experience with HPV, this virus led me to have papilloma's in many parts of my body, I underwent surgeries, chemotherapy, mental and Psychological care and when it seemed that everything was improving there was a problem in my head. In order to determine the nature of the problem, they had to perform a CT scan that showed the presence of a tumor in my head, because, in simple words, fluids dried up on the left side of my brain. On the right side of my head, another condition called idiopathic intracranial hypertension manifested, which was caused by chemotherapy. As you can see, one thing led to another, HPV led me to have precancer, precancer led me to have to have chemotherapy treatments, chemotherapy affected my head with that condition of hypertension, that's why it's important to control HPV in time, because in some cases it can affect your life more than you can imagine. Thank God I am free of HPV, but I am still struggling with the aftermath it left me, although I am still learning to recognize that, no matter what health condition you suffer from, by changing your eating habits you will always be able to improve your health. BECAUSE YOU ARE WHAT YOU EAT.

# Definitions

**HPV** - human papillomavirus.

**Papillomatosis** - is a disorder that is characterized by the presence of numerous papilloma's (warts) on the mucous membranes of the human body.

**Colposcopy** - is a medical diagnostic procedure used to detect cancer cells or abnormal cells that may become cancerous in the cervix, vagina, or vulva.

**Depression** - Illness or mental disorder that is characterized by deep sadness, mood decay, low self-esteem, loss of interest in everything and decreased psychic functions.

**LGBT** - is the acronym composed of the initials of the words **L**esbians, **G**ays, **B**isexual and **T**ransgender. Strictly speaking, its groups people with the sexual orientations and gender identities related to those four words, as well as the communities formed by them.

**Cervix** - the narrow, lower end of the uterus forms a channel between the uterus and vagina.

**pH** – It is the measure of the degree of acidity or alkalinity of a substance or a solution. pH is measured on a scale in the range of 0 to 14. In this range, a pH value of 7 is neutral, which means that the substance or solution is neither alkaline nor acidic. A pH value less than 7 means it is more acidic, and a pH value greater than 7 means it is more alkaline. In medicine, having an appropriate pH in the blood is important for the proper functioning of the body.

**Antiseptic** - These are chemical substances that, applied topically to intact skin, mucous membranes or wounds, reduce or eliminate the population of disease-causing microorganisms.

**Antimicrobial** - are medicines that are used to prevent and treat infections caused by bacteria, viruses, fungi or parasites in humans, animals and plants.

**Vulva** - External genital organs of the woman, including the clitoris, the lips of the vagina, and the opening of the vagina. It is a part of the female reproductive system.

**Stabbing** - sharp pain that feels like a prick.

**CIN1** - slightly abnormal cells found on the surface of the cervix.

**CIN2** - moderately abnormal cells found on the surface of the cervix.

**CIN3** - severely abnormal cells found on the surface of the cervix.

## DEFINITIONS

**RRP** - recurrent respiratory papillomatosis. Rare clinical picture in which wart-like growths called papilloma's form in the airways (in the ducts that connect the nose and mouth to the lungs).

**Tumors** - an abnormal mass of tissue that appears somewhere in the body, caused by an abnormal multiplication of cells.

**Healing** - substance that promotes and accelerates healing.

**Anti-inflammatory** - is the property of a substance or medication that reduces inflammation in the body.

**Antioxidants** - are substances that can protect or slow damage to cells caused by free radicals.

**Regeneration** - is the recovery of a tissue or a part of the body that has been damaged or destroyed.

**Antifungal** - medicine or substance that treats infections caused by fungi.

**Alkaline** - have a pH greater than 7.

**Imbalance** - lack of balance in a situation where the balance between two or more things is not right, fair or equal.

**Immune** system - is a complex network of cells, tissues, organs and the substances they produce that help the body fight infections and other diseases.

**Detoxify** - eliminate in a person the toxic effects that have been caused by harmful or spoiled substances.

**Folic acid** – vitamin B complex nutrient found especially in leafy greens and which the body needs in small amounts to stay healthy.

**Bile** - Fluid produced by the liver and stored in the gallbladder / Term used by Central American Latinos for symptoms attributed to anger or rage including nervous tension, screaming, tremors, gastric dysfunction or, if extreme, unconsciousness.

**Osteoporosis** - a medical condition in which the bones become brittle.

**Chlamydia** – is an infection caused by the bacterium *Chlamydia trachomatis*. It is the most common bacterial sexually transmitted infection worldwide. There are different strains of these bacteria that cause various diseases including trachoma (eye infection), psittacosis, and nonspecific urethritis.

**Gonorrhea** - Gonorrhea is the second most common sexually transmitted infection caused by bacteria worldwide. If left untreated, it can lead to infertility.

**HIV** - also called human immunodeficiency virus. It is the cause of acquired immunodeficiency syndrome (AIDS) and interferes with the body's defense systems responsible for fighting infections and certain types of cancer. The virus can be transmitted through the exchange of certain body fluids of the infected person such as blood, breast milk, semen or vaginal fluids. It is most commonly spread by sexual contact.

**Genital herpes** - a common sexually transmitted infection marked by genital pain and sores.

**Syphilis** - is a bacterial infection that is usually spread by sexual contact. The first stage manifests itself with the appearance of a painless sore (chancre) on the genitals, rectum or mouth. The second stage is the rash on the body that indicates that the virus has already spread. The symptoms then disappear. The third stage is called latent, it can last from 1 to 20 years without experiencing any symptoms. The final stage, which can occur years later can result in damage to the brain nerves, eyes, and heart.

**MONOGAMY** - THE STATE PRACTICE OF BEING MARRIED TO ONLY ONE PERSON. THE PRACTICE OF THE STATE OF HAVING A SEXUAL RELATIONSHIP WITH A SINGLE PARTNER. THE HABIT OF HAVING ONLY ONE PARTNER ATA TIME.

www.ingramcontent.com/pod-product-compliance
Lightning Source LLC
Chambersburg PA
CBHW072251170526
45158CB00003BA/1054